POTENTIALLY DELAY MENOPAUSE

Strategies and Lifestyle Changes to Optimize Your Reproductive Health

DOROTHY LAWSON

TABLE OF CONTENT

INTRODUCTION

I want to start by saying thank you for choosing this book. I hope you found it insightful and helpful.

Understanding Menopause: What to Expect and When

The first chapter of this menopausal book is intended to offer a thorough explanation of what menopause is and what women can expect during this period. It covers a wide range of subjects, such as defining menopause and associated words, the typical age at which menopause begins, the function of hormones in menopause, common menopausal symptoms, the duration of menopause, and the influence of menopause on general health.

Menopause Definition and Related Terms:

Menopause is a normal biological process that occurs when a woman's reproductive years come to an end. It is described as the absence of menstrual cycles for 12 months in a row. Perimenopause is the time before menopause when a woman's hormone levels start to fluctuate and she may experience irregular periods and other symptoms. Postmenopause refers to the years following menopause when a woman's body has finished the hormonal changes associated with menopause.

The Average Age of Menopause Initiation and Factors That Might Influence It:

Menopause often begins at the age of 51. Menopause, on the other hand, can occur at any age, depending on factors such as genetics, lifestyle, and medical conditions. Women who smoke or have had certain medical treatments (such as chemotherapy or radiation therapy) may go through menopause sooner. Women with a family history of early menopause are more likely to go through it themselves.

Hormones' Role in Menopause and Their Effects on the Body:

Hormones, including estrogen, progesterone, and follicle-stimulating hormone, play an important role in menopause. When a woman approaches menopause, her ovaries generate less estrogen and progesterone, causing physiological changes. A reduction in estrogen, for example, might result in vaginal dryness, hot flashes, and other symptoms. During menopause, FSH levels rise, which can lead to hot flashes and other symptoms.

Common Menopausal Symptoms and How They Affect a Woman's Quality of Life:

Typical symptoms of menopause include hot flashes, nocturnal sweats, vaginal dryness, mood changes, and weariness. The severity and length of these symptoms can vary, and they can have a substantial influence on a woman's quality of life. Hot flashes and night sweats, for example, can interrupt sleep and induce irritation, while vaginal dryness might cause pain during sex.

Menopause's Length and What to Expect Throughout Each Stage:

Perimenopause, menopause, and postmenopause are the three stages of menopause. Perimenopause is characterized by fluctuating hormone levels and irregular periods and can extend for several years. Menopause is described as the period-free phase of a woman lasting 12 months. Postmenopause is characterized by hormonal stability and a lower risk of certain health issues and lasts the remainder of a woman's life.

Menopause's Effect on General Health:

Menopause can have a variety of effects on a woman's overall health. Menopause, for example, is linked to an increased risk of osteoporosis, heart disease, and other health problems. Women may, however, take precautions to preserve their health and well-being throughout and beyond menopause.

Menopause's Emotional and Psychological Aspects:

Menopause can have emotional and psychological impacts on women in addition to physical symptoms. Changes in hormone levels, for example, might lead to mood swings, irritation, and anxiety. At this period, women may also suffer changes in their self-image and sexual function.

The Benefits of Delaying Menopause

Delaying menopause has numerous advantages for women. Following are some of the main advantages:

Delaying the start of menopause can help women have more time to conceive: Women might boost their chances of spontaneously conceiving by postponing menopause. This is especially crucial for women who desire to start a family later in life.

Lowering the risk of certain health conditions: The beginning of menopause is linked to a variety of health hazards, including osteoporosis, heart disease, and some malignancies. Women might minimize their risk of these illnesses by postponing menopause.

Increased Quality of Life: Menopause can induce a range of physical and mental symptoms that can severely impair a woman's quality of life. Women might potentially minimize the severity and length of these symptoms by postponing menopause, resulting in a higher quality of life.

Delaying the need for Hormone Replacement Treatment (HRT): HRT is frequently used to treat menopausal symptoms, but it is not without dangers. Women might delay the need for HRT by postponing menopause, limiting their exposure to its hazards.

Maintaining Sexual Function: Menopause can lead to changes in sexual function, such as diminished libido and vaginal dryness. Women might potentially keep their sexual function and sexual health by postponing menopause.

Overall, postponing menopause has a variety of advantages for women, ranging from increased fertility to improved quality of life and lower health risks. It is crucial to remember, however, that not all women may be able to postpone menopause, and that there may be hazards involved with doing so. Any woman considering postponing menopause should speak with her doctor to decide the best course of action.

CHAPTER ONE

LIFESTYLE CHANGES FOR DELAYING MENOPAUSE

Nutrition for Reproductive Health

Nutrition is vital in sustaining reproductive health and increasing the possibility of postponing the onset of menopause. Eating a well-balanced, nutrient-dense diet can help regulate hormones, boost fertility, and promote a healthy pregnancy, all of which can help postpone menopause.

Protein: Is required for the formation and repair of tissues, including reproductive tissues. Protein sources that may be included in a healthy diet include lean meats, seafood, beans, lentils, and nuts.

Iron: This is another important vitamin for reproductive health since it is required for the creation of haemoglobin, which transports oxygen to the body's cells. Iron deficiency can cause anaemia, which can interfere with fertility and pregnancy. Red meat, chicken, fish, beans, lentils, and fortified cereals are all high in iron and can assist promote reproductive health.

Folic Acid: This is essential for the early development of the neural tube, which subsequently develops into the baby's brain and spinal cord. Folic acid-rich foods include leafy green vegetables, citrus fruits, legumes, and fortified grains, which may all be included in a balanced diet.

Calcium: This is a vital nutrient for reproductive health since it is required for healthy bones and teeth, as well as for muscle function and hormone control. Calcium-rich foods include dairy products, leafy green vegetables, and calcium-fortified drinks and cereals.

Omega-3 Fatty Acids: These are necessary for the development of the brain and eyes in fetuses and babies, and they also contain anti-inflammatory effects that can help with fertility and pregnancy. Fatty fish like salmon, walnuts, chia seeds, and flaxseeds are all good sources of omega-3s that may be integrated into a balanced diet.

Vitamin D: Is required for calcium absorption as well as healthy bones and teeth. Sunlight, fortified dairy products, and fatty fish are all good sources of vitamin D, and they can all assist promote reproductive health.

Women can promote their reproductive health and perhaps delay menopause by eating a balanced diel rich in critical nutrients and keeping a healthy weight. It is also critical to minimize your intake of processed and sugary meals, which might have an influence on hormone levels and fertility. Women may enhance their general well-being and maximize their reproductive health by eating a good, balanced diel, perhaps postponing menopause.

Exercise to Improve Reproductive Health

Regular exercise can also help to improve reproductive health and perhaps postpone menopause. Physical activity can assist to manage hormone levels, decreasing stress, and enhancing general health, all of which can improve fertility and pregnancy outcomes. Exercise can help with reproductive health in the following ways:

Hormone Regulation: Exercise can help manage hormone levels such as estrogen and progesterone, which are vital for reproductive health. Frequent physical exercise has been demonstrated to lower estrogen levels in overweight or obese women, which can aid in conception.

Stress Reduction: Stress can have a detrimental influence on fertility and overall reproductive health. Exercise has been demonstrated to lower stress and anxiety, which has been linked to better fertility and pregnancy outcomes.

Keeping a Healthy Weight: Keeping a healthy weight is crucial for reproductive health since being overweight or obese can have a detrimental influence on fertility and pregnancy outcomes. Exercise can aid in the burning of calories and the maintenance of a healthy weight, which can improve fertility and pregnancy outcomes.

Improving Circulation: Frequent exercise helps increase blood flow and circulation to the reproductive organs, which can improve fertility and sexual performance.

Lowering the Risk of Chronic Diseases: Obesity, diabetes, and heart disease can all have a detrimental influence on reproductive health and raise the chance of early menopause. Exercise can help lower the risk of these disorders, promoting reproductive health and perhaps postponing menopause.

Generally, regular exercise can help to improve reproductive health and even postpone menopause. When beginning a new exercise program, it is critical to engage in regular physical activity that is appropriate for your age and fitness level, as well as to talk with a healthcare specialist.

Reproductive Health Stress Management Strategies

Stress may have a severe influence on reproductive health, and studies show that it may also lead to the beginning of menopause at an earlier age. As a result, stress management is a crucial part of potentially postponing menopause and enhancing reproductive health.

Several stress management approaches may be used to relieve tension and enhance relaxation. Mindfulness meditation, which entails focusing on the present moment and accepting it without judgment, is one successful strategy. Frequent mindfulness meditation practice has been demonstrated to lower stress and anxiety while also improving mood and general well-being.

Deep breathing exercises are another strategy that can assist to soothe the body and relieve tension. This entails taking slow, deep breaths and gently exhaling. Deep breathing practice for a few minutes a day can have a big influence on stress levels.

Regular exercise is also an effective stress reliever. Exercise may aid in the release of endorphins, which are natural mood enhancers, as well as improve sleep and general wellness. Regular physical exercises, such as walking, running, yoga, or strength training, can aid in stress reduction and relaxation.

Journaling, talking to a therapist, spending time in nature, practising gratitude, and indulging in hobbies or activities that offer joy and fulfilment are all stress management approaches that may be beneficial.

Stress has been related to irregular periods, infertility, and even early menopause, and it may have a considerable influence on a woman's reproductive health. Prolonged stress can also raise cortisol and other stress hormone levels, which can disturb the body's delicate hormonal balance and interfere with reproductive function.

As a result, stress management practices should be included in your daily routine to promote reproductive health and maybe postpone menopause. Among the effective stress management approaches are:

Mindfulness and meditation can help you decrease stress and anxiety, enhance your sleep, and promote relaxation. Frequent practice can assist you in being more aware of your thoughts and emotions, as well as developing a stronger feeling of inner calm.

Yoga is a mild kind of exercise that can aid with stress reduction, flexibility and strength, and relaxation. It has also been proven to have a favourable influence on hormone levels, including the reduction of cortisol.

Exercise can help decrease stress, boost mood, and improve general health. It can also aid in the maintenance of a healthy weight, which might benefit reproductive health and perhaps postpone menopause.

Deep breathing and diaphragmatic breathing are two breathing practices that can help relieve tension and promote relaxation.

Cognitive-behavioural therapy (CBT): CBT is a type of talk therapy that can assist you in identifying negative thought patterns and developing new stress-management methods.

Integrating these stress-reduction tactics into your daily routine will help lessen the impact of stress on your reproductive health and perhaps postpone menopause.

Reproductive Health Via Sleep Hygiene

A collection of behaviours and activities that support excellent quality sleep is referred to as sleep hygiene. Obtaining adequate quality sleep is critical for reproductive health and may help to postpone menopause. Here are some suggestions for better sleep hygiene:

Stick to a consistent sleep Schedule: Maintain a consistent sleep schedule by going to bed and waking up at the same time every day, especially on weekends.

Create a relaxing bedtime routine: Develop a peaceful evening rouline that includes taking a warm bath, reading a book, or doing some easy stretching exercises to help your body relax and prepare for sleep.

Create a comfortable sleep environment: Establish a relaxing sleeping environment by making your bedroom quiet, dark, and chilly. Get a good mattress and pillows.

Minimize coffee and alcohol consumption: Caffeine and alcohol can disrupt sleep, so try to limit your consumption, especially in the evening.

Avoid using electronic devices before going to bed: The blue light generated by electronic screens might disrupt your body's natural sleep-wake cycle. For at least an hour before going to bed, avoid using phones, tablets, and laptops.

Regular Exercise: can help you manage your body's natural sleep-wake cycle and enhance your sleep quality. Exercise should be avoided too close to bedtime since it might be stimulating.

Control stress: As previously stated, stress can influence sleep quality and reproductive health. Use stress-reduction strategies like deep breathing exercises, meditation, or yoga.

You might potentially postpone menopause and improve general reproductive health by practising excellent sleep hygiene. Obtaining adequate quality sleep is vital for hormone balancing and can help minimize the risk of menopausal health issues including ostcoporosis and cardiovascular disease.

CHAPTER TWO

HORMONE HEALTH AND MENOPAUSE DELAY

Hormone Replacement Therapy

Hormone Replacement Treatment (HRT) is a medical therapy that includes the replacement of hormones that the body no longer produces following menopause. It entails the use of estrogen and progesterone (or synthetic copies of these hormones) to reduce menopausal symptoms and enhance the general quality of life.

HRT may take the form of tablets, patches, gels, or creams, and the precise kind and amount of hormones used will depend on the individual's requirements and medical history. HRT is often prescribed for women who experience severe or incapacitating menopausal symptoms, such as hot flashes, night sweats, and vaginal dryness, and who do not have any contraindications to hormone treatment, such as a history of breast cancer or blood clots.

Although hormone replacement therapy (HRT) may be very helpful in lowering menopausal symptoms and enhancing the quality of life, it is not without dangers. Long-term estrogen usage alone may raise the risk of uterine cancer, while estrogen and progesterone use together can Increase the risk of breast cancer, blood clots, and stroke. As a result, women contemplating HRT should discuss the possible advantages and dangers with their healthcare professionals and carefully monitor any side effects or changes in health status.

ET is generally administered to women who have had a hysterectomy since they no longer have a uterus and so do not need the progesterone component. EPT is recommended for women who still retain their uterus since progesterone protects the uterine lining against cancer.

Menopausal symptoms such as hot flashes, nocturnal sweats, vaginal dryness, and mood swings may be greatly reduced with HRT. Although menopause increases the risk of osteoporosis, it may also help prevent bone loss and minimize the risk of fractures.

HRT, on the other hand, is not without hazards. Long-term HRT usage may raise the risk of some cancers, including breast cancer and endometrial cancer, as well as stroke and blood clots. HRT may also exacerbate pre-existing health issues including high blood pressure and liver disease.

Like with any medical therapy, it is important to examine the possible advantages and dangers of HRT with a healthcare professional to establish whether it is the best decision for a specific person. Women who have a history of breast cancer, blood clots, or stroke may be unsuitable for HRT.

Other therapies for menopausal symptoms, such as natural supplements, lifestyle adjustments, and non-hormonal pharmaceuticals, are available in addition to HRT. To choose the optimal way for treating menopausal symptoms and improving reproductive health, it is important to consider all choices and consult with a healthcare specialist.

Fertility Preservation Methods

Fertility preservation treatments can postpone menopause and sustain reproductive health. These procedures are especially relevant for women who are at risk of experiencing early menopause owing to factors such as cancer treatment or hereditary disorders.

Egg freezing is a frequent fertility preservation procedure. This entails collecting and storing a woman's eggs, which may afterwards be thawed and fertilized if she chose to seek motherhood. Embryo freezing is another approach, which entails fertilizing the eggs with sperm and freezing the resultant embryos.

There are other experimental procedures available, such as ovarian tissue cryopreservation, which involves removing and freezing a part of a woman's ovary before transplanting the tissue back into her body to restore fertility. This approach, however, is still in the experimental stage and may not be generally accessible.

It's vital to remember that fertility preservation methods aren't infallible and don't ensure future conception. They may, however, give an alternative for women who wish to postpone menopause and keep their reproductive choices open.

It's also crucial to examine the dangers and limits of fertility preservation treatments, such as the expense and possible side effects of hormone medicines used to boost egg production in preparation for egg or embryo freezing.

Finally, following a careful assessment of individual circumstances and consultation with a healthcare expert, the choice to undertake fertility preservation treatments should be taken.

Herbal and Natural Reproductive Health Remedies

Herbal and natural therapies might be a good alternative for women who want to improve their reproductive health and perhaps postpone menopause. Although these remedies should not be used in place of medical care, they may be utilized as supplementary treatments to help with reproductive health.

Here are some natural and herbal therapies that may be useful:

Black Cohosh: This is a herb that has long been used to treat hot flashes and other menopausal symptoms. It may also aid in the regulation of menstrual periods.

Dong Quai: Dong Quai is a traditional Chinese medicine herb used to regulate menstrual cycles and treat menstrual cramps. It may potentially have estrogenic properties in the body.

Maca: This is a root vegetable that has traditionally been used in traditional medicine to boost fertility and libido. It may also assist to alleviate menopausal symptoms.

Vitex: Vitex, commonly known as chaste berry, is a herb that has traditionally been used to regulate menstrual cycles and ease premenstrual syndrome symptoms (PMS). It may also aid with fertility.

Red Clover: Red clover includes isoflavones, which have estrogen-like actions in the body. It may assist to alleviate menopausal symptoms such as hot flashes.

Evening Primrose Oil: Evening primrose oil is high in gamma-linolenic acid (GLA), which may help balance hormone levels and alleviate PMS symptoms.

Flaxseed: Flaxseed is a plant-based source of omega-3 fatty acids, lignans, and phytoestrogens, which may aid with hormone regulation and reproductive support.

Red Raspberry Leaf: The herb red raspberry leaf is often used to enhance menstrual health and conception. It may also assist with PMS and menopausal symptoms.

It is crucial to remember that herbal and natural therapies might have negative effects and combine with other prescriptions, so consult with your doctor before taking them. Moreover, although some studies have revealed that these therapies may be beneficial to reproductive health, additional study is required to completely understand their effects.

CHAPTER THREE

REPRODUCTIVE HEALTH OPTIMIZATION

Menopause and Sexual Health

Menopause may have serious consequences for a woman's sexual health. The drop in estrogen levels that occurs after menopause may result in a loss in vaginal lubrication, weakening of the vaginal tissues, and a decrease in flexibility, all of which can cause pain during sexual activity. These modifications may potentially raise the risk of vaginal and urinary tract infections.

Menopause may influence a woman's emotional and psychological health, as well as her sexual desire and pleasure, in addition to physical changes. Women, for example, may suffer mood swings, melancholy, and anxiety throughout menopause, which might influence their sexual attraction.

Thankfully, there are several techniques available to assist control these symptoms and maintain sexual health throughout menopause. To alleviate pain during sexual activity, one way is to use vaginal lubricants or moisturizers. Hormone replacement treatment (HRT) may also assist with vaginal dryness and other menopausal symptoms that affect sexual health.

Regular physical exercise is another technique that might help decrease stress and enhance mood. Exercise has also been demonstrated to boost female sexual function.

Communication with sexual partners is essential for sustaining a successful sexual connection throughout menopause, in addition to physical and behavioural changes. Communication about sexual wants and preferences that is open and honest may assist promote closeness and happiness.

Overall, sexual health is an essential element of menopausal reproductive health. Women may maintain a full and pleasurable sex life during this period of transition by taking efforts to control physical symptoms, promote mental well-being, and maintain good relationships.

Keeping Your Bones Healthy During Menopause

A woman's body goes through hormonal changes throughout menopause, which may cause bone loss and raise her risk of osteoporosis. Keeping bone healthy at this period is critical for avoiding fractures and being healthy overall. Here are some tips for keeping your bones healthy throughout menopause:

Calcium and Vitamin D Intake: Calcium is essential for healthy bones, while vitamin D is required for calcium absorption. Calcium-rich foods include dairy products, leafy green vegetables, and calcium-fortified drinks and cereals. Sunlight exposure and fortified dairy products are two sources of vitamin D. Women over the age of 50 should consume 1200mg of calcium and 800 IU of vitamin D every day.

Exercise regularly: Walking, running, and weight lifting are all weight-bearing workouts that may help develop and maintain bone density. Exercise also helps to improve balance and coordination, which may help to reduce falls and fractures.

Stop smoking: It has been shown that smoking increases the risk of osteoporosis and bone fractures. Smoking cessation may help prevent bone loss and enhance overall health.

Reduce Alcohol Consumption: Excessive alcohol use has been related to bone loss and increased fracture risk. Ladies should restrict themselves to one drink each day.

Consider the following medication: If a woman is at high risk for osteoporosis, her doctor may advise her to take bone-building medicine. Bisphosphonates and hormone treatment, for example, may help maintain bone density and minimize the risk of fractures.

Regular bone density testing may help identify bone loss early, allowing for early management to avoid future bone loss.

It is critical to maintaining bone health throughout menopause for general health and well-being. Women may avoid bone loss and fractures by implementing these methods into their everyday practice.

Keeping Your Mental Wellness Alive Throughout Menopause

Menopause is a big life shift that may have serious consequences for a woman's mental health. At this period, it is typical for women to suffer worry, despair, mood changes, and irritability. Women, on the other hand, may take precautions to preserve their mental health and deal with these changes.

Prioritizing self-care is a crucial component. This may include participating in relaxing activities such as meditation, yoga, or deep breathing techniques. Exercise regularly may also assist to boost mood and decrease stress.

It is also critical to have a solid support system. This might include discussing your situation with friends or family members, as well as joining a support group for women going through menopause. Therapy might also be beneficial for people who need more organized assistance.

Medication may be required in certain circumstances to treat symptoms of sadness or anxiety. To choose the appropriate course of therapy, women should explore their choices with their healthcare physician.

It's also critical for women to remain involved in activities they like and to pursue their interests. This may assist to offer a feeling of purpose and satisfaction, which is especially crucial during times of change.

Ultimately, sustaining mental health throughout menopause entails a mix of self-care, support, and, when required, seeking professional assistance. Women may better traverse this stage of life and emerge with a higher feeling of well-being if they take these measures.

CHAPTER FOUR

CONCLUSION

Empowering Yourself to Delay Menopause: Bringing It All Together

Using a comprehensive approach to potentially delaying menopause includes lifestyle modifications, diet, exercise, stress management, and maybe even medical therapies such as hormone replacement therapy or fertility preservation methods. Here are some ideas to help you bring it all together:

Examine your current way of life: Examine your present habits and routines objectively. Are you getting enough exercise? Are you consuming a nutritious, well-balanced diet? Are you getting enough quality sleep? Are you handling stress effectively? Determine where you can make good adjustments.

Change your diet: Integrate the critical nutrients covered previously in this article into your diet. Eat a variety of nutritious meals while limiting processed and sugary items.

Exercise regularly: Participate in regular physical activity that incorporates both cardiovascular and strength training.

Reduce stress: Find stress-reduction methods that work for you, such as meditation, yoga, or deep breathing exercises.

Consider hormone replacement therapy: If you are having severe menopausal symptoms and other treatments have failed, talk to your healthcare practitioner about the potential of hormone replacement therapy.

Consider fertility preservation techniques: If you want to postpone menopause to protect your fertility, talk to your doctor about your choices.

Prioritize your mental health: Practice self-care, remain socially engaged, and get help if necessary to preserve your mental health.

You might postpone menopause and preserve your general well-being by adopting a complete approach to your reproductive health. It is crucial to talk with your healthcare physician before making any substantial lifestyle changes or contemplating medical procedures.

www.ingramcontent.com/pod-product-compliance
Lightning Source LLC
Chambersburg PA
CBHW061557250726
48657CB00021B/2078